The Glowing Guide

GLOW UP!

Achieving Beautiful Skin through Holistic Skincare

Violet Jackson

TABLE OF CONTENTS

INTRODUCTION

In our modern world, it's no secret that skincare has become a multi-billion-dollar industry. With countless products promising to transform our skin and give us that coveted "glow," it's easy to feel overwhelmed and unsure of where to start.

Enter The Glowing Guide: Achieving Beautiful Skin through Holistic Skincare. This book is not just another skincare manual; it aims to revolutionise the way we think about and approach skincare. Instead of focusing solely on external products and quick fixes, this guide takes a holistic approach, emphasising the importance of nourishing our skin from within and considering all aspects of our lifestyle that can impact its health and appearance.

In the introduction, we explore the benefits of this holistic approach to skincare. By understanding the interconnectedness of our body, mind, and skin, we can unlock the secrets to achieving true radiance and lasting beauty. We also delve into the importance of consistency and patience, as we learn that skincare is a journey rather than a destination.

Throughout the book, we guide readers through the different chapters, each one tackling a different aspect of holistic skincare. We start with Chapter One, where we help readers identify their unique skin type and understand its specific needs. From there, we dive into addressing common skin concerns such as acne, ageing, and hyperpigmentation, providing targeted solutions and expert advice.

Chapter Two focuses on nourishing our skin from within, highlighting the crucial role that diet plays in skin health. We explore the nutrients and supplements that can enhance our skin's radiance, and provide practical tips for incorporating them into our daily lives.

Chapter Three is all about creating an effective skincare routine. We teach readers how to choose the right products for their specific skin type and concerns and emphasise the importance of proper cleansing, exfoliation, and moisturization. With the right routine, we can maximise the benefits of our products and achieve our skincare goals.

In Chapter Four, we showcase special treatments that can take our skincare game to the next level. From DIY masks and facial treatments that can be done at home to professional treatments that should be considered, we cover it all. With these insights, we can pamper our skin and give it the extra care it deserves.

In Chapter Five, we go beyond skincare and explore the lifestyle factors that impact our skin. We delve into the effects of stress and sleep on our skin health, and highlight the importance of sun protection and safe skin care practices. By understanding these factors, we can make informed choices that promote our overall well-being and radiance.

In conclusion, we summarise our journey towards sustainable skin health and a glowing complexion. We offer final thoughts and tips for readers as they continue their skincare journey, armed with the knowledge and tools provided in this guide.

So, if you're ready to transcend the surface-level approach to skincare and achieve beautiful skin from within, join us on this transformative journey. The Glowing Guide is here to empower you with the knowledge and insight needed to unlock your skin's true potential. Your radiant complexion awaits.

The Benefits of a Holistic Approach to Skincare

A holistic approach to skincare offers numerous benefits that can greatly contribute to achieving and maintaining healthy, radiant skin. By recognizing that our skin is not an isolated entity, but rather a reflection of our overall well-being, we can unlock the potential for true transformation and long-lasting results. Let us delve into some of the key advantages of adopting a holistic approach to skincare:

1. Addresses the Root Cause: Unlike many conventional skincare methods that focus solely on superficial symptoms, a holistic approach seeks to identify and address the root cause of skin concerns. Instead of simply treating a breakout or dry skin, it explores underlying factors such as diet, lifestyle, stress, and hormonal imbalances that may be contributing to these issues. By addressing the root cause, holistic skincare tackles the problem at its source, leading to more sustainable and effective results.

2. Nourishes Skin from Within: Holistic skincare recognizes the vital role that nutrition plays in skin health. It emphasises the consumption of

wholesome, nutrient-dense foods that provide the necessary vitamins, minerals, antioxidants, and fatty acids to nourish the skin from within. By focusing on a balanced diet that includes fruits, vegetables, healthy fats, and lean proteins, we can support optimal skin health and promote a clear, glowing complexion.

3. Minimises Toxic Exposure: Many conventional skincare products contain a multitude of harmful ingredients, such as synthetic fragrances, parabens, sulphates, and phthalates. These chemicals can disrupt the skin's natural balance, clog pores, and even contribute to long-term health problems. The holistic approach prioritises using natural, organic, and non-toxic skincare products, reducing our exposure to harmful substances and supporting the skin's natural processes.

4. Promotes Mind-Body Connection: Holistic skincare recognizes the intimate connection between our mental and emotional well-being and our skin health. Stress, anxiety, and lack of sleep can manifest on our skin in the form of breakouts, dullness, and inflammation. By incorporating stress management techniques, such as meditation, yoga, or mindfulness practices into our daily routine, we can promote a healthy mind-body connection and indirectly improve our skin health.

5. Embraces Self-Care Rituals: A holistic skincare approach encourages self-care rituals that go beyond the application of products. It emphasises the importance of taking time for ourselves, engaging in activities that bring joy and relaxation, and finding moments of tranquillity amidst our busy lives. By prioritising self-care, we reduce stress levels and create an overall sense of well-being, which can positively impact our skin health.

6. Personalised Approach: Holistic skincare recognizes that every individual's skin is unique, and what works for one person may not work for another. It encourages customization and empowers individuals to understand their specific skin concerns, needs, and preferences. By tailoring skincare routines and products specifically to their skin type and concerns, individuals can optimise their results and achieve a healthy, well-balanced complexion.

Incorporating a holistic approach to skincare can lead to transformative benefits that extend far beyond a glowing complexion. By embracing this approach, individuals can experience improved overall well-being, increased self-confidence, and a deeper connection to their bodies. It allows us not only to care for our skin but also to cultivate a more profound sense of self-love and acceptance, leading to a positive ripple effect in all aspects of our lives.

The Importance of Consistency and Patience

Consistency and patience are two essential components when it comes to achieving beautiful skin through a holistic skin care approach. While instant results may be desirable, embracing a long-term perspective and committing to a consistent routine are vital for attaining and maintaining healthy, radiant skin. Here's why consistency and patience matter in the realm of holistic skincare:

1. Skin Renewal Process: Our skin has a natural renewal process that takes time. It typically takes about four to six weeks for new skin cells to surface from the deeper layers and replace the old ones at the surface. By maintaining a consistent skincare routine, we ensure that our skin receives the necessary care and nourishment throughout this process, promoting healthy cell turnover and revealing fresh, youthful skin over time.

2. Balancing the Skin: Consistency is key in creating a stable environment for our skin. By regularly following a holistic skincare routine, we support our skin's natural balance and optimise its overall health. This includes cleansing, exfoliating, moisturising, and protecting the skin using natural and effective products tailored to our specific needs. Consistency allows the skin to adapt and respond positively to the chosen skincare regimen, helping to regulate oil production, reduce inflammation, and improve overall skin tone and texture.

3. Addressing Concerns Over Time: Some skin concerns, such as hyperpigmentation, acne, or wrinkles, require time and consistency to be adequately addressed. Holistic skincare takes a holistic, long-term approach to resolving these concerns. By consistently using targeted ingredients, such as vitamin C for brightening or retinol for anti-aging, we enable the skin to gradually improve over time. Patience is essential, as visible results may take weeks or even months to manifest, but the results achieved through this approach tend to be more sustainable and lasting.

4. Building Healthy Habits: Consistency in skincare extends beyond the products we use. It also involves adopting healthy lifestyle habits that contribute to overall skin health. This includes

maintaining a balanced diet, staying hydrated, managing stress levels, getting adequate sleep, and protecting the skin from harmful environmental factors like UV rays. By integrating these habits into our daily lives and consistently adhering to them, we create a holistic approach that supports skin health from the inside out.

5. Preventing Skin Damage: Consistency in holistic skincare is not only about addressing existing skin concerns but also about preventing future damage. By consistently using sunscreen and practising sun protection measures, we shield our skin from harmful UV radiation, which is a major contributor to premature ageing, pigmentation issues, and skin cancer. Over time, consistent sun protection can significantly reduce the appearance of sun damage and promote a youthful complexion.

6. Developing a Mindful Relationship with Skin: Consistency and patience in holistic skincare foster a mindful relationship with our skin. By slowing down, observing, and listening to our skin's needs, we become more in tune with its changing conditions. This allows us to make adjustments to our routine when necessary and respond appropriately to any imbalances or concerns that arise. A mindful approach also helps us appreciate

progress and small improvements along the way, leading to increased self-care and self-love.

Ultimately, consistency and patience in holistic skincare practice provide the foundation for achieving beautiful, healthy skin. By investing in a routine that considers the unique needs of our skin, we effectively nurture its inherent healing abilities and gradually witness the positive results unfold. Embracing a long-term perspective and cultivating patience allow us to experience the true transformative power of holistic skincare for lifelong skin health and radiance.

CHAPTER 1

Skin Types and Concerns

There are various skin types and concerns that individuals may face, each requiring specific care and attention. Understanding these different skin types and concerns can guide us in choosing the right skincare products and routines to address specific needs. Here are some common skin types and concerns:

1. Normal Skin:
Normal skin is characterised by a balanced moisture level, small pores, and an even skin tone. People with normal skin often have minimal concerns and can typically tolerate a wide range of skincare products. However, maintaining a consistent skincare routine is still essential to preserve the skin's health and clarity.

2. Dry Skin:
Dry skin lacks moisture and often feels tight, rough, or flaky. It may appear dull and may be more prone to fine lines and wrinkles. The primary concern for individuals with dry skin is to hydrate and nourish the skin deeply. Using moisturisers with hydrating ingredients such as hyaluronic acid and oils can

14

help restore moisture and strengthen the skin's barrier.

3. Oily Skin:

Oily skin results from excessive sebum production, leading to a shiny complexion and enlarged pores. Those with oily skin may have a higher risk of developing acne and blackheads. The main concern for oily skin is to control excess oil and maintain a balanced complexion. Using gentle, oil-free cleansers and products with ingredients like salicylic acid can help regulate oil production and keep pores clear.

4. Combination Skin:

Combination skin refers to having both oily and dry areas on the face. Typically, the T-zone (forehead, nose, and chin) is oilier, while the cheeks may be drier. Balancing hydration while controlling oil can be a challenge for individuals with combination skin. Using products formulated for combination skin or targeting specific areas accordingly can help maintain a harmonious balance.

5. Sensitive Skin:

Sensitive skin is easily irritated, often exhibiting redness, itching, or a burning sensation in response to certain products or environmental factors. It requires gentle and soothing skincare to avoid exacerbating sensitivity. Products formulated without harsh ingredients like fragrance, alcohol, or dyes, along with patch-testing new products, can help alleviate sensitivity and reduce potential reactions.

6. Ageing Skin:

Ageing skin experiences a natural decline in collagen and elastin production, leading to the formation of wrinkles, sagging, and loss of firmness. Improving the signs of ageing generally involves promoting collagen production and providing intense hydration. Skincare products with antioxidants, retinol, peptides, and hyaluronic acid can help stimulate cell turnover, improve elasticity, and diminish the appearance of fine lines and wrinkles.

7. Hyperpigmentation:

Hyperpigmentation refers to areas of darkened skin caused by an overproduction of melanin. It can be a result of sun damage, hormonal changes, acne scars, or skin inflammation. Addressing hyperpigmentation often involves the regular use of brightening agents, such as vitamin C, niacinamide, or hydroquinone, along with a diligent sun protection routine to prevent further damage.

8. Acne-Prone Skin:

Acne-prone skin is characterised by frequent breakouts, including pimples, blackheads, and whiteheads. It may result from excess oil production, clogged pores, bacteria, or hormonal factors. Treating acne-prone skin usually involves gentle cleansing, along with the use of non-comedogenic products, exfoliating ingredients like salicylic acid, and possibly topical treatments prescribed by a dermatologist.

By identifying your specific skin type and concerns, you can tailor your skincare routine to address them effectively. Remember, seeking professional advice from a dermatologist when dealing with severe skin conditions or persistent concerns is advisable for proper diagnosis and treatment.

Identifying Your Skin Type and Understanding its Needs

Understanding the needs of different skin types is essential for maintaining a healthy and balanced complexion. Let's delve into each skin type in more detail and explore the specific needs they have:

1. Dry Skin:

Dry skin lacks moisture and tends to feel tight, itchy, and sometimes even rough or flaky. The primary need for dry skin is hydration. Look for skincare products that are rich in emollients, humectants, and occlusive ingredients to provide intense moisture and lock it in. Ingredients like hyaluronic acid, glycerin, shea butter, and ceramides work wonders for dry skin. Avoid harsh cleansers or drying exfoliants that strip away natural oils and choose gentle, creamy formulas instead.

2. Oily Skin:

Oily skin is characterised by excess sebum production, resulting in a shiny complexion, enlarged pores, and the tendency to develop acne or blackheads. The key needs for oily skin are oil control and pore refinement. Opt for oil-free or lightweight products that regulate oil production without causing dryness. Gentle exfoliation is crucial to keep the pores clear, but avoid overdoing it, as excessive scrubbing can lead to more oil production. Look for ingredients like salicylic acid, niacinamide, and clay to help control excess oil and minimise pores.

3. Combination Skin:

Combination skin is a mix of oily and dry areas, with the T-zone (forehead, nose, and chin) often being oilier and the cheeks drier. The needs of combination skin involve finding a balance between hydration and oil control. Use lightweight, oil-free moisturisers to hydrate dry areas without exacerbating oiliness. Targeted treatments are beneficial for addressing specific concerns in various regions of the face, such as using mattifying products in the oilier areas and richer moisturisers in the drier patches.

4. Normal Skin:

Normal skin is well-balanced and generally doesn't have any major concerns. However, it still requires regular care to maintain its health and prevent issues. The primary needs for normal skin are hydration, protection from environmental factors, and general maintenance. Choose moisturisers with a balanced formula that provide adequate hydration without being heavy or greasy. Incorporate products with antioxidants, such as vitamins C and E, to protect the skin from free radicals and maintain its youthful appearance.

5. Sensitive Skin:

Sensitive skin is easily irritated and may react to certain ingredients or external factors. Understanding the needs of sensitive skin involves gentle and soothing care. Look for products that are free from fragrance, alcohol, and harsh chemicals. Opt for gentle cleansers, hypoallergenic moisturisers, and physical sunscreens instead of chemical ones. Calming ingredients like aloe vera, chamomile, and oat extract can help soothe and protect sensitive skin.

Additionally, all skin types benefit from a few universal needs. These include regular cleansing to remove dirt, excess oil, and impurities, as well as protection from the sun's harmful UV rays by applying broad-spectrum sunscreen daily. Exfoliation is essential for all skin types to shed dead skin cells and promote a smoother, brighter complexion. However, the frequency and type of exfoliation may vary depending on the skin's sensitivity and needs.

Remember that everyone's skin is unique, and your needs may differ even within the defined skin types. Regularly assess your skin's condition and adjust your skincare routine accordingly. Consulting with a dermatologist can be helpful in determining your skin type and developing a personalised skincare regimen to address specific concerns.

Addressing Common Skin Concerns

Addressing common skin concerns requires a targeted approach to effectively treat and manage specific issues. Here, we will discuss some of the most common skin concerns and offer guidance on how to address them:

1. Acne:

Acne is a prevalent skin concern that occurs when hair follicles become clogged with oil, dead skin cells, and bacteria. To address acne, it's crucial to establish a consistent skincare routine:

- Cleanse the skin twice a day with a gentle, non-comedogenic cleanser to remove dirt and excess oil.
- Use products containing ingredients like salicylic acid or benzoyl peroxide, which help unclog pores and reduce inflammation.
- Avoid picking or squeezing pimples, as this can lead to further infection and scarring.
- Moisturize with lightweight, oil-free moisturisers to maintain hydration without exacerbating oiliness.
- Consider spot treatments or topical creams prescribed by a dermatologist to target stubborn breakouts.
- In severe cases, oral medications or professional treatments like chemical peels or light therapy may be necessary.

2. Hyperpigmentation:

Hyperpigmentation refers to the darkening or discoloration of certain areas of skin, resulting from increased melanin production. To address hyperpigmentation:

- Protect your skin from sun exposure by applying broad-spectrum sunscreen with a high SPF on a daily basis.
- Incorporate topical treatments that contain ingredients like hydroquinone, retinoids, vitamin C, or azelaic acid, which help fade pigmentation and even out skin tone.
- Exfoliate regularly to promote cell turnover and fade hyperpigmentation. Chemical exfoliants like alpha-hydroxy acids (AHAs) or beta-hydroxy acids (BHAs) can be beneficial.
- Consider professional treatments like chemical peels, microdermabrasion, or laser therapy for more severe or resistant cases.

3. Dryness/Dehydration:
Dryness and dehydration can result in tight, flaky, and itchy skin. To address these concerns:

- Hydrate the skin from within by drinking an adequate amount of water daily.
- Use a gentle, hydrating cleanser that doesn't strip away natural oils.

- Moisturize regularly with a rich, emollient moisturiser to restore and retain moisture.
- Apply facial oils or serums containing ingredients like hyaluronic acid, glycerin, or ceramides to lock in moisture.
- Avoid long, hot showers or baths, as they can strip the skin of essential oils.
- Consider using a humidifier to add moisture to the air in drier environments.

4. Sensitivity/Redness:
Sensitive skin often experiences redness, irritation, and discomfort. To address sensitivity and redness:

- Avoid using harsh, fragranced, or irritating products. Opt for gentle, hypoallergenic formulations.
- Patch test new products before applying them to your face, especially if you have sensitive skin.
- Use mild, non-foaming cleansers that won't disrupt the skin's natural barrier.
- Moisturize with soothing creams or lotions containing ingredients like aloe vera, chamomile, or oat extract.
- Protect your skin by wearing sunscreen with physical blockers like zinc oxide or titanium dioxide.

- Consult with a dermatologist if your sensitivity or redness persists, as it may indicate an underlying condition such as rosacea or eczema.

It's important to remember that consistent and patient skincare routines are key to addressing and managing common skin concerns. Results may take time, and what works for one person may not work for another. If your concerns persist or worsen, seeking professional advice from a dermatologist or skincare specialist is highly recommended. They can provide personalised recommendations and treatments tailored to your specific needs.

CHAPTER 2

Nourishing Your Skin From Within

Nourishing your skin from within is an essential aspect of maintaining healthy, radiant skin. While external skincare products and treatments are beneficial, taking care of your skin internally can have a profound impact on its overall health and appearance. Here are some key ways to nourish your skin from within:

1. Hydration:
One of the simplest yet most crucial steps in nourishing your skin is staying hydrated. Drinking an adequate amount of water throughout the day helps flush out toxins, improves circulation, and maintains optimal skin function. Aim to drink at least eight glasses (64 ounces) of water daily, and increase your intake during periods of intense physical activity or in hot weather.

2. Balanced Diet:
Eating a balanced and nutritious diet plays a significant role in nourishing your skin. Include the following key nutrients in your meals:

- Antioxidants: Found in fruits and vegetables, antioxidants help protect the skin against free radicals, which can cause premature ageing. Incorporate colourful produce such as berries, leafy greens, citrus fruits, and tomatoes into your diet.

- Omega-3 Fatty Acids: These healthy fats are essential for maintaining skin health and reducing inflammation. Sources include fatty fish like salmon and mackerel, walnuts, flaxseeds, and chia seeds.

- Vitamins and Minerals: Consume foods rich in vitamins A, C, E, and zinc. Vitamin A helps regulate skin cell production, vitamin C promotes collagen synthesis, vitamin E protects against UV damage, and zinc aids in wound healing. Foods like carrots, sweet potatoes, oranges, broccoli, almonds, and pumpkin seeds are excellent sources.

3. Reduce Inflammatory Foods:

Certain foods can exacerbate inflammation in the body, leading to skin issues like acne, redness, or sensitivity. Limit your consumption of processed foods, sugary snacks, refined carbohydrates, and foods high in saturated fats. Instead, opt for whole foods, lean proteins, and healthy fats to reduce inflammation and support overall skin health.

4. Protect Your Skin from the Sun:

Excessive sun exposure can lead to premature ageing, pigmentation, and increase the risk of skin cancer. Shield your skin from the harmful effects of UV rays by wearing sunscreen daily with at least SPF 30. Additionally, seek shade during peak sun hours and wear protective clothing, a wide-brimmed hat, and sunglasses.

5. Manage Stress:
Chronic stress can contribute to a variety of skin concerns, including acne breakouts, eczema flare-ups, or dull complexion. Find healthy ways to manage stress, such as practising meditation or mindfulness, engaging in regular exercise, getting enough sleep, and pursuing activities that bring you joy. Also, consider incorporating stress-reducing practices like yoga or deep breathing exercises into your routine.

6. Adequate Sleep:
Proper sleep is essential for overall health and skin rejuvenation. During sleep, the body repairs and regenerates cells, including skin cells. Aim for 7-8 hours of quality sleep each night to allow your skin time to replenish and restore.

7. Regular Exercise:
Engaging in regular physical activity boosts blood circulation, which nourishes the skin by delivering oxygen and vital nutrients. Exercise also promotes the elimination of toxins through sweat,

contributing to a healthier complexion. Choose activities you enjoy, whether it's brisk walking, cycling, dancing, or any other form of exercise that gets you moving.

Remember, nourishing your skin from within is a holistic approach that works in synergy with external skincare routines. By adopting a healthy lifestyle, focusing on hydration, a balanced diet, sun protection, stress management, quality sleep, and regular exercise, you can enhance your skin's vitality and achieve a radiant, healthy complexion.

The Role of Diet in Skin Health

Nourishing your skin from within starts with understanding the role of diet in skincare. The food you consume has a direct impact on the health and appearance of your skin. By making conscious choices about what you eat, you can enhance your skin's natural radiance and support its overall well-being. Here's a detailed exploration of the role of diet in skincare:

1. Collagen Production:
Collagen is a protein that provides structure and elasticity to the skin. As we age, the natural production of collagen decreases, leading to fine

lines, wrinkles, and sagging skin. However, you can support collagen production through your diet. Certain foods are rich in nutrients that promote collagen synthesis, such as vitamin C, amino acids, and antioxidants. Include foods like citrus fruits, bell peppers, berries, leafy greens, tomatoes, avocado, and bone broth in your diet to support collagen formation and maintain skin elasticity.

2. Antioxidants:

Antioxidants are essential for protecting the skin from damage caused by free radicals, which are unstable molecules that can harm healthy cells. Free radicals are generated by factors like pollution, ultraviolet (UV) radiation, and stress. Antioxidant-rich foods help neutralise free radicals and reduce oxidative stress in the body. Include colourful fruits and vegetables, such as berries, spinach, kale, carrots, and sweet potatoes, which are packed with antioxidants like vitamins A, C, and E.

3. Hydration:

Proper hydration is vital for healthy skin. When your body is well-hydrated, it helps maintain the skin's moisture barrier, preventing dryness, flakiness, and irritation. Drinking an adequate amount of water throughout the day also supports the body's detoxification process, helping flush out toxins that can lead to skin issues. In addition to water, consume hydrating foods like cucumbers, watermelon, oranges, and celery, which have high water content.

4. Healthy Fats:
Healthy fats are crucial for maintaining supple and moisturised skin. Omega-3 fatty acids, in particular, are well-known for their anti-inflammatory properties and ability to nourish the skin. These fats help reduce skin inflammation, prevent dryness, and support skin barrier function. Sources of omega-3 fatty acids include fatty fish like salmon, mackerel, and sardines, as well as plant-based sources like flaxseeds, chia seeds, and walnuts.

5. Low-Glycemic Index Foods:
High-glycemic index foods, such as refined carbohydrates, sugary snacks, and processed foods, can contribute to skin problems like acne and inflammation. They rapidly increase blood sugar levels, leading to insulin spikes, which may stimulate oil production and inflammation in the skin. Opt for low-glycemic index foods, including whole grains, legumes, leafy greens, and lean proteins, to help maintain more stable blood sugar levels and promote clear skin.

6. Vitamins and Minerals:

A balanced diet rich in vitamins and minerals can have a significant impact on your skin's health. Vitamin A plays a crucial role in skin cell production and renewal. Find it in foods like carrots, sweet potatoes, and leafy greens. Vitamin C supports collagen synthesis and can be obtained from citrus fruits, peppers, and berries. Vitamin E helps protect the skin from environmental damage and is found in foods like almonds, sunflower seeds, and spinach. Zinc, another essential mineral, aids in wound healing and can be found in oysters, pumpkin seeds, and lean meats.

7. Gut Health:
The health of your gut microbiome, the collection of bacteria in your digestive system, influences your overall well-being, including your skin. A healthy gut contributes to improved nutrient absorption and metabolism, which can positively impact your skin's appearance. Consuming probiotic-rich foods like yoghurt, sauerkraut, kimchi, and kefir can help support a healthy gut, leading to improved skin health.

Learning to nourish your skin from within is an ongoing journey. Incorporating a balanced diet that includes nutrient-rich foods, hydrating adequately, and making conscious choices about your food intake can go a long way in supporting your skin's health and radiance. Keep in mind that everyone's skin is unique, so it may take time to determine which foods work best for you. Additionally, consulting with a dermatologist or a registered dietitian can provide personalised guidance tailored to your specific skin care needs.

Nutrients and Supplements for Radiant Skin

Achieving radiant skin goes beyond topical skincare products. Nourishing your skin from within with the right nutrients and supplements can enhance its natural glow and overall health. Here, we will delve into the essential nutrients and supplements that promote radiant skin:

1. Omega-3 Fatty Acids:
Omega-3 fatty acids are beneficial fats that help maintain skin hydration, reduce inflammation, and enhance skin elasticity. These healthy fats can be found in fatty fish like salmon, mackerel, and sardines, as well as plant-based sources such as flaxseeds, chia seeds, and walnuts. If incorporating enough omega-3s into your diet is challenging, you may consider omega-3 supplements derived from fish oil or algae.

2. Vitamins A, C, and E:

Vitamin A, also known as retinol, plays a vital role in skin cell production and renewal. It promotes a healthy complexion, reduces the appearance of fine lines and wrinkles, and supports normal oil production. Sources of vitamin A include carrots, sweet potatoes, leafy greens, and liver. However, excessive vitamin A intake can be toxic, so consider consuming it through food rather than supplementation.

Vitamin C is a powerful antioxidant that supports collagen synthesis, helping to maintain skin elasticity and combat the signs of ageing. It also aids in protecting the skin from UV damage and brightening the complexion. Citrus fruits, berries, peppers, and leafy greens are excellent sources of vitamin C. You may also consider vitamin C supplements for an additional boost.

Vitamin E is another potent antioxidant that helps protect the skin from free radicals and environmental damage. It supports skin repair and moisturization, promoting a youthful appearance. Nuts, seeds, spinach, and avocados are rich in vitamin E. While supplementation is an option, it's important to consult a healthcare professional to determine the appropriate dosage.

3. Collagen Peptides:
Collagen is a protein that provides structure and elasticity to the skin. As we age, natural collagen production declines. Supplementing with collagen peptides can help replenish and support collagen production, promoting skin firmness and reducing the appearance of wrinkles. Collagen supplements are available in various forms, including powders, capsules, and liquid formulations. Ensure you choose a high-quality, hydrolyzed collagen supplement for optimal absorption and effectiveness.

4. Hyaluronic Acid:
Hyaluronic acid is a molecule that helps retain moisture within the skin, keeping it plump, hydrated, and smooth. It can be found in skincare products but can also be taken orally as a supplement. Hyaluronic acid supplements can enhance skin moisture levels and improve the appearance of fine lines and wrinkles. When selecting a hyaluronic acid supplement, opt for a reputable brand and follow the recommended dosage.

5. Antioxidants:
Antioxidants are essential for neutralising free radicals that damage skin cells and accelerate

ageing. They protect the skin from environmental stressors and help maintain a youthful complexion. Besides vitamins A, C, and E mentioned earlier, other antioxidants include selenium, zinc, and green tea extract. Consuming a diet rich in fruits, vegetables, nuts, and seeds can ensure you're getting an array of antioxidants. If needed, consult with a healthcare professional to determine if antioxidant supplements are necessary for your skin health.

Remember, while supplements can support radiant skin, they work best when combined with a healthy, balanced diet. Additionally, it's crucial to consult a healthcare professional or a registered dietitian before starting any new supplements, as they can guide you on appropriate dosages and potential interactions with medications. Alongside proper nutrition, practising good skincare habits and protecting your skin from sun exposure are also essential for maintaining a radiant complexion.

CHAPTER 3

Creating an Effective Skincare Routine

In order to achieve and maintain beautiful and healthy skin, it is imperative to establish an effective skincare routine that suits your specific needs. A well-designed skincare routine can transform your complexion, address specific concerns, and promote overall skin health. This chapter of "The Glowing Guide: Achieving Beautiful Skin through Holistic Skincare" explores the key elements of an effective skincare routine and provides guidance on how to choose the right products for your skin type and concerns.

1. Cleansing:
Cleansing is the foundation of any skincare routine. It removes dirt, excess oil, impurities, and pollutants that accumulate on the skin's surface throughout the day. Choosing the right cleanser for your skin type is crucial. Foaming cleansers are ideal for oily and combination skin, while cream or gel cleansers are better suited for dry or sensitive skin. It is important to cleanse your face twice a day, once in the

morning and once in the evening, to maintain a clean and balanced complexion.

2. Exfoliation:

Exfoliation is a step that should not be overlooked in your skincare routine. It helps to remove dead skin cells, unclog pores, and promote cell turnover, resulting in smoother and brighter skin. There are two types of exfoliation: physical and chemical. Physical exfoliants use a scrub or brush to physically remove dead skin cells, while chemical exfoliants use ingredients like alpha-hydroxy acids (AHAs) or beta-hydroxy acids (BHAs) to dissolve and remove dead skin cells. It is important to exfoliate 2-3 times a week, depending on your skin's tolerance, to avoid over-exfoliation and irritation.

3. Moisturization:

Moisturizing is a crucial step in any skincare routine, regardless of your skin type. Moisturisers replenish hydration, lock in moisture, and create a protective barrier on the skin to prevent moisture loss. For oily or acne-prone skin, choose lightweight, oil-free, or gel-based moisturisers that won't clog pores. Dry or mature skin can benefit from richer, cream-based moisturisers that provide deep hydration. It is important to moisturise your skin twice a day, after cleansing, to ensure optimal hydration and maintain a healthy skin barrier.

4. Sun Protection:
Protecting your skin from the harmful effects of the sun is a non-negotiable step in your skincare routine. Sun exposure can lead to premature ageing, sunburn, hyperpigmentation, and even skin cancer. Choose a broad-spectrum sunscreen with an SPF of 30 or higher and apply it generously to all exposed areas of your skin. It is crucial to reapply sunscreen every two hours, especially when spending extended periods outdoors. For added protection, consider using a moisturiser or foundation with built-in SPF.

5. Targeted Treatments:
To address specific skin concerns such as acne, ageing, or hyperpigmentation, incorporate targeted treatments into your skincare routine. These treatments usually come in the form of serums, ampoules, or spot treatments that contain potent active ingredients. Retinol, vitamin C, niacinamide, hyaluronic acid, and AHAs are some examples of effective ingredients for specific concerns. It is important to introduce one new treatment at a time to assess its effectiveness and monitor your skin's reaction.

6. Eye Care:

The delicate skin around the eyes requires extra care and attention. Incorporate an eye cream or gel into your skincare routine to address concerns such as dark circles, puffiness, and fine lines. Look for ingredients like caffeine, peptides, hyaluronic acid, and vitamin K that help to reduce puffiness, hydrate, and improve the appearance of the under-eye area. Apply the eye cream using your ring finger, gently tapping it onto the skin to avoid tugging or pulling.

7. Consistency and Patience:

Consistency is key when it comes to skincare. It can take time for your skin to adjust to a new skincare routine and for you to see noticeable results. Be patient and give your skin at least a month to adapt to the new products and ingredients. Avoid switching products frequently, as this can disrupt your skin's balance and result in further irritation or breakouts. Stick to the routine and give it time to work its magic.

When creating an effective skincare routine, it is essential to understand and listen to your skin's unique needs. Pay attention to how your skin reacts to certain products and adjust accordingly. Remember that achieving healthy, glowing skin is a journey, and consistency, along with the right products and techniques, will help you achieve your desired results. With the knowledge and guidance provided in this chapter, you can create a personalised skincare routine that will nurture and transform your skin.

Choosing the Right Products for Your Skin Type and Concerns

Choosing the right skincare products is vital to address your specific skin type and concerns effectively. With countless options available on the market, it can be overwhelming to navigate through the sea of products and find the ones that are best suited for your skin. In this chapter of "The Glowing Guide: Achieving Beautiful Skin through Holistic Skincare," we will explore how to choose the right products for your skin type and concerns, ensuring that you make informed decisions and achieve optimal results.

1. Determine Your Skin Type:
Before selecting any skincare products, it is essential to identify your skin type. The four main skin types are oily, dry, combination, and sensitive. Oily skin is characterised by excess sebum production and often appears shiny and prone to

breakouts. Dry skin lacks moisture, feels tight, and may appear flaky or rough. Combination skin has both oily and dry areas, typically with an oily T-zone (forehead, nose, and chin) and drier cheeks. Sensitive skin is easily irritated, reactive, and may have redness or itching. Understanding your skin type will help you choose products specifically formulated to cater to its unique needs.

2. Consider Your Skin Concerns:

Apart from your skin type, it is important to identify specific concerns you want to address. Whether it be acne, ageing, hyperpigmentation, or sensitivity, there are products available that target and improve these conditions. Look for key ingredients that are known to be effective for your specific concerns. For example, salicylic acid and benzoyl peroxide are commonly used to treat acne, while retinol and peptides are beneficial for anti-aging concerns. Understanding your concerns will narrow down your choices and allow you to select products that will truly make a difference.

3. Read and Understand Product Labels:

To choose the right products, it is crucial to read and understand product labels. Pay attention to the ingredients listed and their concentrations. Ingredients are often listed in descending order based on their concentration in the product. Look for products that have active ingredients listed higher up in the list, as they are more likely to have a significant impact. Avoid products that contain potentially harmful ingredients such as parabens, sulphates, artificial fragrances, and alcohol, as they can cause irritation or allergic reactions. Opt for products with natural and organic ingredients, as they are generally gentler on the skin.

4. Perform Patch Tests:

Performing patch tests before incorporating new products into your routine is a crucial step to avoid potential adverse reactions. Apply a small amount of the product to a small patch of skin, usually on the jawline or behind the ear, and observe for any signs of irritation or allergic reactions over a 24 to 48-hour period. If there are no adverse reactions, it is usually safe to proceed with using the product on your entire face. Patch tests are especially important for those with sensitive or reactive skin.

5. Seek Professional Advice:

If you find it overwhelming to choose the right products for your skin type and concerns, consider seeking advice from skincare professionals. Dermatologists, estheticians, or even knowledgeable skincare consultants at beauty stores can provide valuable insight and recommendations based on your specific needs. They can assess your skin, identify your concerns, and suggest suitable products or ingredients that will address your unique needs effectively.

6. Start with a Basic Routine:
When first starting a skincare routine or introducing new products, it is best to keep it simple and gradually build up. Begin with a basic routine consisting of a gentle cleanser, moisturiser, and sunscreen that are appropriate for your skin type. Once your skin has adjusted to this basic routine, you can gradually incorporate additional products such as exfoliants, serums, or masks to address specific concerns. Slowly introducing new products allows you to monitor how your skin reacts and ensures that you do not overload your skin with too many new ingredients at once.

7. Take Note of Your Skin's Response:
After incorporating new products into your routine, pay close attention to how your skin responds. Monitor for any signs of irritation, redness, breakouts, or increased sensitivity. If you notice any negative reactions, discontinue use of the product immediately. On the other hand, if you see positive changes such as improved texture, reduced blemishes, or increased hydration, continue using the product and adjust your routine accordingly.

Choosing the right products for your skin type and concerns is a process that requires careful consideration and experimentation. By understanding your skin type, identifying your concerns, reading product labels, performing patch tests, seeking professional advice when needed, and paying attention to your skin's response, you can create a skincare routine tailored to your specific needs. Remember that skincare is not one-size-fits-all, and what works for someone else may not work for you. With patience and persistence, you will be able to curate a skincare regimen that nurtures and transforms your skin, helping you achieve the healthy and radiant complexion you desire.

The Importance of Proper Cleansing, Exfoliation, and Moisturization

Proper cleansing, exfoliation, and moisturization are the foundation of any effective skincare routine. These three steps play a crucial role in maintaining healthy, radiant skin and addressing various skin concerns. In this chapter of "The Glowing Guide: Achieving Beautiful Skin through Holistic Skincare," we will discuss in detail the significance of proper cleansing, exfoliation, and moisturization, and how they contribute to the overall health and appearance of your skin.

1. Cleansing:

Cleansing your skin is the first and most essential step in any skincare routine. It helps remove dirt, oil, makeup, environmental impurities, and dead skin cells that accumulate throughout the day. By keeping your skin clean, you prevent clogged pores, breakouts, and dullness. Proper cleansing also prepares your skin to absorb subsequent skincare products more effectively.

When choosing a cleanser, consider your skin type and specific concerns. For oily or acne-prone skin, a gel or foaming cleanser that helps control excess oil and unclog pores is recommended. Dry or sensitive skin types may benefit from gentle, creamy cleansers that hydrate and soothe the skin. It is important to cleanse your skin twice daily, once in the morning and once in the evening, to ensure optimal cleanliness and to remove any impurities that may have accumulated overnight.

2. Exfoliation:

Exfoliation is a vital step in achieving a smooth, even complexion. It involves removing the buildup of dead skin cells on the surface of your skin, revealing a fresh layer underneath. Regular exfoliation promotes cell turnover, enhances skin radiance, and improves the absorption of other skincare products. It can also help prevent clogged pores, blackheads, and acne breakouts.

There are two types of exfoliation: physical and chemical. Physical exfoliation involves using a scrub or brush to physically remove dead skin cells. Chemical exfoliation, on the other hand, involves using products with specific ingredients like alpha-hydroxy acids (AHAs) or beta-hydroxy acids (BHAs) that dissolve the bonds between dead skin cells, allowing them to be sloughed off more easily.

It is crucial to choose the appropriate exfoliation method for your skin type and concerns. Physical exfoliation may be too harsh for sensitive or acne-prone skin, while chemical exfoliation can be gentler and more effective for those with these concerns. It is generally recommended to exfoliate 1-3 times per week, depending on your skin's tolerance and needs.

3. Moisturization:
Moisturization is key to maintaining healthy, hydrated skin. It replenishes the moisture barrier, protects the skin from environmental damage, and helps lock in hydration. Regardless of your skin type, moisturization is essential to balance oil

production, prevent dryness, and keep your skin looking plump and youthful.

When selecting a moisturiser, consider your skin type and specific concerns. For oily or acne-prone skin, look for lightweight, oil-free formulations that provide hydration without clogging pores. Dry or mature skin benefits from richer, more emollient moisturisers that nourish and hydrate the skin. It is important to apply moisturiser after cleansing and exfoliating, both morning and night, to ensure your skin stays moisturised throughout the day.

Additionally, don't overlook the importance of using a moisturiser with SPF during the day. Sun protection is a crucial aspect of skincare to prevent premature ageing, sunburns, and skin damage caused by UV rays. Choose a broad-spectrum sunscreen with an appropriate SPF level for your daily needs.

In summary, proper cleansing, exfoliation, and moisturization are fundamental steps in any skincare routine for maintaining healthy and vibrant skin. Cleansing removes impurities, exfoliation eliminates dead skin cells, and moisturization nourishes and hydrates the skin. By incorporating these steps into your daily skincare regimen, you can achieve optimal skin health, address specific concerns, and enjoy a radiant complexion. Remember that consistency and using products suitable for your skin type and concerns are key to maximising the benefits of these skincare steps.

CHAPTER FOUR

Treating Your Skin to Special Treatments

While a regular skincare routine of cleansing, exfoliating, and moisturising forms the foundation of healthy skin, there are times when our skin needs extra care and attention. Special treatments go beyond the basics and allow us to address specific concerns, target problem areas, and enhance the overall health and appearance of our skin. In this chapter of "The Glowing Guide: Achieving Beautiful Skin through Holistic Skincare," we delve into the importance and benefits of treating your skin to special treatments.

1. Face Masks:
Face masks are an excellent way to provide targeted treatment for various skin concerns. They come in different forms, including clay masks, sheet masks, gel masks, and cream masks, each with its unique benefits. Face masks are designed to deliver concentrated ingredients to the skin, providing hydration, detoxification, brightening, or clarifying effects.

Clay masks, for example, are fantastic for purifying the skin by drawing out impurities and excess oil. They can be especially beneficial for those with oily or acne-prone skin. On the other hand, sheet masks are soaked in serum that tends to provide intense hydration and nourishment to the skin. Gel masks are known for their cooling and soothing properties, making them suitable for sensitive or irritated skin. Cream masks are typically rich in moisturising ingredients and are ideal for dry or dehydrated skin.

Incorporating face masks into your skincare routine can provide a spa-like experience, rejuvenate your skin, and address specific concerns. Depending on your needs, you can use face masks once or twice a week or whenever your skin requires a boost of hydration or a targeted treatment.

2. Serums:
Serums are potent, concentrated treatments packed with active ingredients that address specific skin concerns. They typically have a lightweight, fast-absorbing texture that allows the ingredients to penetrate deeper into the skin. Serums come in various formulations, targeting issues such as hydration, brightening, anti-aging, and acne.

For example, hyaluronic acid serums are excellent for boosting hydration and plumping the skin, making them suitable for dry or dehydrated skin types. Vitamin C serums are known for their brightening and antioxidant properties, helping to reduce hyperpigmentation and promote a more even skin tone. Retinol serums, on the other hand, work on reducing the appearance of fine lines, wrinkles, and promoting cellular turnover. A variety of serums are available, and choosing the right one for your specific concerns can bring significant benefits to your skincare routine.

Serums are generally applied after cleansing and toning and should be followed by a moisturiser to seal in the active ingredients. Due to their potency, apply only a few drops of serum and gently massage it into the skin. Depending on the serum and your skin's tolerance, they can be used daily or a few times a week.

3. Facial Treatments:
Facial treatments, such as facials, chemical peels, microdermabrasion, and laser therapies, are professional-grade procedures performed by trained estheticians or dermatologists. These treatments provide deeper and more intensive care for your skin, targeting specific concerns and achieving more significant results.

Facials are customised treatments that typically involve a combination of cleansing, exfoliation, extractions, masks, and massages. They provide deep cleansing, hydration, and rejuvenation for the skin, leaving it refreshed and glowing. Peels involve applying a solution to the skin to remove the outermost layer, revealing smoother, brighter skin underneath. They can address issues like hyperpigmentation, acne scars, and fine lines. Microdermabrasion is a mechanical exfoliation technique that uses a handheld device to remove dead skin cells and improve skin texture. Laser therapies, such as laser resurfacing or laser hair removal, utilise intense light energy for various skincare concerns.

Facial treatments offer more advanced and precise solutions, making them ideal for addressing specific skin issues or achieving significant improvements. They generally require professional assistance and may have different recommended frequencies, depending on the treatment and your skin's needs. Consultation with a skincare professional is highly advisable before undergoing any facial treatment.

Treating your skin to special treatments provides targeted care, addresses specific concerns, and enhances the overall health and appearance of your skin. Face masks, serums, and professional facial treatments go beyond the basics of skincare and offer advanced solutions for various skin needs. Incorporating these special treatments into your routine can provide a boost of nourishment, hydration, and targeted treatment, helping you achieve the beautiful, healthy skin you desire. Remember to choose treatments that are suitable for your skin type, and always consult with a skincare professional for guidance and advice.

DIY Masks and Facial Treatments for Glowing Skin

Achieving a healthy, glowing complexion doesn't always require a trip to the spa or salon. With a little creativity and some kitchen staples, you can create effective DIY masks and facial treatments right at home. In this chapter of "The Glowing Guide: Achieving Beautiful Skin through Holistic Skincare," we explore the world of DIY masks and facial treatments, providing you with natural, affordable options to enhance your skin's radiance.

1. DIY Face Masks:
Creating your own face masks allows you to tailor the ingredients to your specific skin concerns and preferences. Natural ingredients found in your

pantry or refrigerator can provide numerous benefits. Here are a few popular DIY face mask recipes:

a. Honey and Yogurt Mask:
Honey acts as a humectant, drawing moisture to the skin, while yoghurt soothes and exfoliates. Mix one tablespoon of honey with two tablespoons of plain yoghurt and apply to your face. Leave it on for 15-20 minutes before rinsing with warm water. This mask is ideal for all skin types and promotes hydration and a healthy glow.

b. Oatmeal and Banana Mask:
The combination of oatmeal and banana is perfect for calming sensitive or irritated skin. Mash one ripe banana and add three tablespoons of oatmeal. Mix until it forms a paste and apply to your face. Leave it on for 15-20 minutes, then rinse off with lukewarm water. This mask helps soothe inflammation and provides nourishment to your skin.

c. Turmeric and Coconut Oil Mask:
Turmeric is renowned for its antioxidant and anti-inflammatory properties, while coconut oil offers hydration and moisture. Mix one teaspoon of turmeric powder with two

teaspoons of coconut oil until well combined. Apply the mixture to your face and neck, leaving it on for 10-15 minutes. Rinse off gently with warm water. This mask brightens the complexion and promotes overall skin health.

d. Avocado and Honey Mask:
Avocado is packed with essential fatty acids that nourish and hydrate the skin, while honey adds antimicrobial and clarifying properties. Mash half of a ripe avocado and mix it with one tablespoon of honey. Apply the mixture to your face and leave it on for 15-20 minutes before rinsing off with lukewarm water. This mask helps to moisturise, soften, and brighten the skin.

e. Coffee Grounds and Yogurt Mask:
Coffee grounds offer gentle exfoliation, while yoghurt helps to clarify and tighten the skin. Combine one tablespoon of finely ground coffee with two tablespoons of plain yoghurt. Gently massage the mixture onto your face in circular motions for a minute or two, then leave it on for 10-15 minutes. Rinse off with warm water, and follow with your preferred moisturiser. This mask helps

to slough off dead skin cells, improve circulation, and give the skin a radiant glow.

f. Papaya and Lemon Juice Mask:
Papaya contains natural enzymes that break down dead skin cells and promote cellular turnover, while lemon juice brightens and tightens the skin. Mash a small piece of ripe papaya and mix it with one teaspoon of freshly squeezed lemon juice. Apply the mixture to your face and neck, being careful to avoid the eye area. Leave it on for 10-15 minutes, then rinse off with cool water. This mask helps to reveal a fresh, youthful complexion.

Remember to patch test any DIY mask on a small area of skin before applying it to your entire face to ensure you won't experience any adverse reactions. Additionally, these masks are generally safe for most skin types but may not be suitable for those with specific allergies or sensitivities. Always consult with a dermatologist if you have any concerns.

2. DIY Facial Treatments:
In addition to masks, you can also create DIY facial treatments that provide similar benefits to

professional-grade procedures. Here are a few examples:

a. Steam Facial:
Steaming is a simple yet effective way to open up your pores, allowing for a deeper cleanse. Boil water and pour it into a large bowl, carefully positioning your face over the bowl. Drape a towel over your head, creating a tent to trap the steam. Keep your face in the steam for 5-10 minutes, then pat your skin dry and proceed with your usual skincare routine. This treatment helps to remove impurities and improves circulation.

b. Sugar Scrub:
A sugar scrub is an excellent way to exfoliate and remove dead skin cells, leaving your skin smooth and radiant. Mix two tablespoons of sugar (white or brown) with enough olive oil or coconut oil to create a paste. Gently massage the mixture onto damp skin in circular motions for a few minutes, then rinse off with warm water. Follow with your favourite moisturiser. This treatment is suitable for all skin types and can be used once or twice a week.

c. Green Tea Toner:

Green tea is packed with antioxidants and has anti-inflammatory properties, making it an ideal natural toner. Brew a cup of green tea and let it cool. Transfer the tea to a spray bottle and spritz it onto your face after cleansing. Allow it to dry naturally or gently pat it into your skin. This toner can soothe and hydrate the skin and can be used daily.

d. Aloe Vera Gel Soothing Mask:
Aloe vera gel has soothing and cooling properties, making it perfect for calming irritated and inflamed skin. Simply apply a thin layer of pure aloe vera gel onto cleansed skin and leave it on for 15-20 minutes before rinsing off with cool water. This treatment helps to reduce redness, heal blemishes, and promote a healthy, glowing complexion.

e. Bentonite Clay Detoxifying Mask:
Bentonite clay is renowned for its ability to draw out impurities, toxins, and excess oil from the skin. Mix one tablespoon of bentonite clay with enough water to form a thick paste. Apply it to your face, avoiding the eye area, and let it sit for 10-15 minutes or until it's dry. Rinse off with warm water and moisturise afterward. This mask helps to

detoxify the skin, minimise pores, and promote a clearer, more radiant complexion.

f. Cucumber Eye Treatment:
Cucumber is known for its cooling and hydrating properties, making it great for rejuvenating tired or puffy eyes. Slice a cucumber into thin rounds and place them over your closed eyes, allowing them to rest for 10-15 minutes. Alternatively, you can blend cucumber and strain the juice, then soak cotton pads in the juice and place them over your eyes. This treatment helps to reduce puffiness, alleviate dark circles, and refresh the under-eye area.

DIY masks and facial treatments offer a cost-effective and convenient way to pamper your skin and achieve a healthy, radiant complexion. However, it's essential to remember that everyone's skin is unique, and what works for one might not work for another. It's always wise to conduct a patch test on a small area of skin and observe any reactions before applying the treatment to your entire face. Additionally, if you have any pre-existing skin conditions or concerns, it's best to consult with a dermatologist before trying any DIY facial treatments.

DIY masks and facial treatments can help you achieve glowing skin without breaking the bank. From homemade masks customised to your specific needs to simple yet effective at-home treatments, there are plenty of options to suit your skin type and concerns. Take the time to discover and experiment with different ingredients and techniques, but always remember to prioritise the health and safety of your skin.

Professional Treatments: What to Expect and When to Consider

When it comes to achieving glowing, healthy skin, professional treatments can provide a significant boost by targeting specific skin concerns and offering more advanced solutions than what DIY home remedies can achieve. Whether you're dealing with stubborn acne, signs of ageing, uneven skin tone, or simply want to pamper yourself with a luxurious spa experience, there are various professional treatments available to address your specific needs. In this extensive guide, we will explore different types of professional treatments, what to expect during the procedures, and when it may be time to consider seeking professional help.

1. Facial Treatments:

a. Professional Facials:
Professional facials are a popular choice for maintaining healthy skin and targeting specific concerns. During a professional facial, an esthetician will cleanse, exfoliate, extract impurities, perform facial massage, apply masks, and provide personalised skincare recommendations. They may also incorporate techniques like steam, high-frequency stimulation, or LED therapy to enhance results. Professional facials can improve the appearance of your skin, leaving it refreshed, revitalised, and glowing.

b. Microdermabrasion:
Microdermabrasion is a non-invasive exfoliating procedure that involves using a handheld device to gently remove the outermost layer of dead skin cells, revealing smoother, more radiant skin underneath. The treatment can help with issues such as dullness, fine lines, mild acne scars, and uneven texture. It may cause some mild redness or sensitivity temporarily, but there is minimal downtime involved.

c. Chemical Peels:

Chemical peels are effective for addressing various skin concerns, such as acne, hyperpigmentation, fine lines, and sun damage. During a chemical peel, a solution containing exfoliating agents, such as alpha-hydroxy acids (AHAs) or beta-hydroxy acids (BHAs), is applied to the skin. This causes controlled damage that prompts the skin to regenerate, revealing a smoother, more youthful complexion. The intensity of the peel can vary, with some requiring little to no downtime, while others involve a longer recovery period.

2. Advanced Skin Treatments:

a. Laser Treatments:

Laser treatments utilise concentrated light energy to target specific skin concerns. They can be used for various purposes, including hair removal, skin resurfacing, scar reduction, and treatment of hyperpigmentation. Laser treatments can be more invasive compared to other procedures, but advancements in technology have made them more precise, safe, and effective. The results and downtime associated with laser treatments can vary depending on the type and intensity of the laser used.

b. Microneedling:
Microneedling, also known as collagen induction therapy, involves using a device equipped with tiny needles to create controlled micro-injuries on the skin. These micro-injuries stimulate the production of collagen and elastin, leading to skin rejuvenation and improvement in texture, tone, and firmness. Microneedling is effective for treating acne scars, fine lines, wrinkles, and enlarged pores. Depending on the depth of the treatment, redness and mild swelling may occur for a few days post-procedure.

c. Radiofrequency Treatments:
Radiofrequency (RF) treatments use energy waves to heat the deeper layers of the skin, stimulating collagen production and tightening loose or sagging skin. RF treatments are popular for reducing wrinkles, tightening skin, and improving overall skin texture. They are often used in combination with other treatments or as part of a larger anti-aging regimen.

3. Injectable Treatments:

a. Botox:

Botox, a brand name for a neurotoxic protein called botulinum toxin, is used to temporarily relax muscles that cause wrinkles and fine lines. It is commonly used on forehead lines, crow's feet, and frown lines between the eyebrows. Botox injections are relatively quick, with minimal discomfort, and require no downtime. Results typically last for a few months before additional treatments are needed.

b. Dermal Fillers:

Dermal fillers are gel-like substances that are injected beneath the skin to restore volume, fill in wrinkles, and enhance facial contours. Popular dermal fillers contain hyaluronic acid, a naturally occurring substance in the body that provides hydration and plumpness. Different types of dermal fillers can be used for various areas of the face, such as nasolabial folds, lips, and cheeks. The duration of results depends on the type of filler used, with some lasting several months to a year or more.

4. When to Consider Professional Treatments:

While DIY home remedies and skincare routines can help maintain healthy skin, there are certain instances where seeking professional treatments may be beneficial:

a. Persistent Skin Concerns:
If you've been dealing with persistent skin issues like severe acne, deep scarring, chronic redness, or hyperpigmentation that do not improve with over-the-counter treatments, professional intervention can provide more targeted and effective solutions.

b. Special Occasions:
If you have an upcoming special event, like a wedding or a milestone celebration, professional treatments can help you achieve a radiant and flawless complexion in a shorter time frame. Treatments like facials, chemical peels, or laser rejuvenation can refresh your skin and boost your confidence.

c. Ageing Concerns:
As we age, our skin goes through natural changes, including the loss of collagen, thinning skin, and the appearance of fine lines and wrinkles. Professional treatments

such as Botox, fillers, or skin tightening procedures can help address these concerns and restore a more youthful appearance.

d. Desire for Professional Expertise:
Sometimes, seeking professional treatments is simply a choice to benefit from the expertise and knowledge of licensed professionals. Estheticians and dermatologists can assess your skin, provide personalised recommendations, and customise treatments according to your specific needs and goals.

e. Self-care and Pampering:
Lastly, professional treatments provide an opportunity for self-care, relaxation, and pampering. Enjoying a facial, a massage, or a full-body spa treatment can help alleviate stress, improve overall well-being, and give you a much-needed break from your daily routine.

It's important to note that not all professional treatments are suitable for everyone. It's always recommended to consult with a licensed professional, such as an esthetician or dermatologist, who can evaluate your skin condition, medical history, and unique needs before recommending any specific treatments.

Professional treatments offer a wide range of skincare solutions that can address various concerns, from basic skin maintenance to more advanced anti-aging procedures. Depending on your goals and specific skin needs, there are facial treatments, advanced skin treatments, and injectable options available. When DIY remedies and routine skincare regimens fail to produce desired results, or on special occasions when you want to look your absolute best, considering professional treatments can provide the extra boost that your skin needs for a healthy, glowing complexion.

CHAPTER 5

Beyond Skincare: Lifestyle Factors that Impact Your Skin

Maintaining healthy and radiant skin goes beyond simply adhering to a skincare routine. While the products and treatments you use on your skin play a crucial role, several lifestyle factors can significantly impact the overall health and appearance of your skin. In this article, we will explore some of these factors and how they can influence your skin's condition.

1. Diet: The foods you consume have a direct impact on your skin health. A diet rich in fruits, vegetables, whole grains, and lean proteins provides essential nutrients and antioxidants that promote healthy skin. On the other hand, a diet high in processed foods, sugary snacks, and unhealthy fats can lead to inflammation, acne breakouts, and premature ageing. It is important to maintain a balanced diet and stay hydrated to support optimal skin health.

2. Hygiene: Proper hygiene practices can contribute to maintaining clear and healthy skin. Regularly

washing your face and body with gentle cleansers helps remove dirt, sweat, and excess oil that can clog pores and lead to breakouts. However, over-washing or using harsh cleansers can strip the skin of its natural oils, causing dryness and irritation. Find a balance and tailor your skincare routine to your skin type and individual needs.

3. Sun Exposure: Overexposure to the sun's harmful ultraviolet (UV) rays is one of the leading causes of skin damage and premature ageing. UV radiation can penetrate the skin, leading to sunburns, pigmentation irregularities, wrinkles, and even skin cancer. It is crucial to protect your skin from the sun by using broad-spectrum sunscreen with a high SPF, seeking shade during peak sunlight hours, and wearing protective clothing and accessories like hats and sunglasses.

4. Stress: Chronic stress can wreak havoc on your skin. When you are under stress, your body releases cortisol, a hormone that triggers inflammation and can exacerbate skin conditions such as acne, eczema, and psoriasis. Stress can also disrupt your sleep patterns and negatively impact the skin's ability to repair and regenerate. Engaging in stress-reducing activities like exercise, meditation, and self-care practices can help improve your skin's health.

5. Sleep: Getting sufficient quality sleep is essential for overall health, and your skin is no exception. During sleep, your body repairs and regenerates cells, including your skin cells. Inadequate or poor-quality sleep can impair this regenerative process, leading to a dull complexion, under-eye circles, and an increased likelihood of skin issues. Aim for 7-9 hours of uninterrupted sleep each night to support your skin's rejuvenation.

6. Smoking and Alcohol Consumption: Smoking and excessive alcohol consumption can have detrimental effects on your skin. Smoking restricts blood vessels, reducing blood flow to the skin and depleting it of oxygen and nutrients. This can cause the skin to appear dull, wrinkled, and aged. Alcohol dehydrates the body, including the skin, leading to dryness and inflammation. It can also exacerbate conditions like rosacea and acne.

7. Environmental Factors: Environmental factors such as pollution and harsh weather conditions can take a toll on your skin. Air pollution can increase oxidative stress and trigger inflammation, leading to skin damage and various skin concerns. Additionally, extreme temperatures, wind, and low humidity can cause dryness, redness, and irritation. Taking protective measures like using barrier

creams, wearing appropriate clothing, and using air purifiers can help mitigate these effects.

8. Exercise: Regular physical activity not only benefits your overall health but also has positive effects on your skin. Exercise increases blood circulation, which delivers oxygen and nutrients to your skin cells, promoting a healthy, glowing complexion. Sweating during exercise helps to unclog pores and cleanse the skin. However, it is important to cleanse your skin afterward to remove any sweat and bacteria to avoid potential breakouts.

9. Hormonal Changes: Hormonal fluctuations throughout life can have a significant impact on your skin. Puberty, menstruation, pregnancy, and menopause are all stages when hormonal changes can result in various skin concerns. Increased hormonal activity can stimulate oil production, leading to acne breakouts. It's important to adapt your skincare routine to these changing hormonal needs and consider seeking professional advice if necessary.

10. Medications: Certain medications can cause side effects that affect the skin. For example, some medications, including birth control pills and antibiotics, can disrupt the natural balance of bacteria in the gut, leading to skin imbalances such

as acne or fungal infections. If you notice any changes in your skin coinciding with starting a new medication, consult with your healthcare provider to discuss any potential underlying causes and solutions.

11. Allergens and Irritants: Exposing your skin to allergens and irritants can trigger allergic reactions, irritations, and skin conditions such as eczema or contact dermatitis. Common allergens and irritants include certain cosmetics, fragrances, detergents, and certain chemical ingredients. Identifying and avoiding these triggers can help minimise skin issues and maintain a healthy complexion.

12. Sleep Position: Believe it or not, the position in which you sleep can impact your skin's health. Sleeping on your stomach or side can lead to the formation of sleep lines and wrinkles, as well as the potential for increased breakouts. The repeated pressure on the skin can cause collagen breakdown over time. It is recommended to sleep on your back to minimise contact between your face and the pillow, reducing the potential for skin ageing and breakouts.

13. Emotional Well-being: Mental and emotional well-being can reflect on your skin. Stress, anxiety, and depression can lead to increased inflammation,

hormonal imbalances, and compromised immune function, all of which can manifest as various skin problems. Practising stress management techniques, seeking therapy if needed, and engaging in activities that promote emotional well-being can help maintain healthy skin.

14. Skincare Habits: Beyond the actual skincare products, your skincare habits can impact your skin's health. Over-exfoliation, aggressive scrubbing, and using harsh products can strip the skin of its natural oils, disrupt the skin barrier, and lead to dryness, redness, and irritation. It is important to be gentle with your skin, choose suitable products for your skin type, and follow a consistent routine that includes cleansing, moisturising, and protecting your skin.

Combining a comprehensive skincare routine with these lifestyle factors is key to achieving healthy and radiant skin. Identifying any potential triggers or habits that may negatively impact your skin and making the necessary adjustments can go a long way in maintaining the overall health and appearance of your skin. Remember, everyone's skin is unique, so be observant and adapt your lifestyle choices accordingly to support your individual skin health. Healthy skin starts from within, so nourish your body and mind to achieve your best skin.

The Role of Stress and Sleep in Skin Health

Stress and sleep play significant roles in skin health. Let's dive deeper into each of these factors:

Stress:
1. Inflammation: When the body is under stress, it releases stress hormones like cortisol. Elevated cortisol levels can lead to increased inflammation, which can trigger or exacerbate numerous skin conditions such as acne, eczema, psoriasis, and rosacea.

2. Oil Production: Stress also influences sebaceous gland activity, leading to an overproduction of oil. This excess oil can clog pores, contributing to the formation of acne breakouts.

3. Impaired Skin Barrier Function: Chronic stress weakens the skin's natural barrier function, making it more vulnerable to environmental aggressors and moisture loss. This can result in dryness, redness,

and a compromised skin barrier that is less effective at retaining moisture and protecting against irritants.

4. Delayed Wound Healing: Stress can impede the body's ability to heal wounds. High-stress levels interfere with the production of collagen, a crucial protein for wound healing, leading to slower recovery times and potentially leaving scars or marks on the skin.

5. Skin Ageing: Chronic stress promotes premature ageing through a process called glycation. Excess cortisol levels can accelerate the breakdown of collagen and elastin, contributing to the development of wrinkles, fine lines, and sagging skin.

6. Impaired Immune Function: High levels of stress weaken the immune system, making the skin more susceptible to infection and inflammation. This can lead to conditions such as acne, cold sores, and even exacerbate conditions like psoriasis and eczema.

7. Skin Sensitivity: Stress can heighten skin sensitivity, making it more reactive to external irritants. This can result in redness, itching, and increased discomfort for individuals with conditions like rosacea or sensitive skin.

8. Altered Skin Microbiome: Stress affects the balance of the skin's microbiome, which is the community of microorganisms that live on the skin's surface. Disruptions to the microbiome can contribute to imbalances in the skin, leading to conditions like acne and dermatitis.

9. Hair and Nail Health: Chronic stress can lead to hair loss or thinning, as stress hormones can disrupt the hair growth cycle. Stress can also impact the strength and appearance of nails, making them brittle and more prone to breakage.

To manage stress and support skin health, consider incorporating stress-management techniques into your routine. This may include practices such as exercise, meditation, deep breathing exercises, mindfulness, yoga, and engaging in activities that bring joy and relaxation. Additionally, seeking support from friends, family, or professionals can be valuable in managing stress levels and improving overall well-being.

Sleep:
1. Skin Repair and Renewal: During sleep, the body undergoes significant repair and regeneration processes. This includes the skin, which uses this time to repair any damage incurred throughout the day. Adequate sleep allows for optimal cell

turnover, collagen production, and tissue repair, resulting in healthier, more youthful-looking skin.

2. Circulation and Blood Flow: Quality sleep promotes proper blood circulation, ensuring the delivery of oxygen and nutrients to the skin cells. This improved circulation can contribute to a more radiant complexion.

3. Dark Circles and Puffiness: Lack of sleep can lead to the formation of dark circles, fine lines, and puffiness around the eyes. Sleep deprivation causes the blood vessels under the thin skin around the eyes to dilate, resulting in a tired and aged appearance.

4. Hormonal Balance: Sleep deprivation disrupts hormonal balance, causing increases in stress hormones like cortisol. These hormonal imbalances can directly contribute to various skin issues, including acne breakouts and inflammation.

5. Increased Skin Regeneration: During sleep, the body goes into a state of repair and regeneration. Skin cells regenerate and repair the damage caused by environmental factors like UV radiation. Sufficient sleep allows for this essential rejuvenation process, leading to healthier and more youthful-looking skin.

6. Moisture Balance: While we sleep, our body boosts hydration levels and repairs the skin's moisture barrier. Proper hydration is critical for maintaining supple and hydrated skin. Inadequate sleep can disrupt this process, resulting in dryness and a compromised skin barrier.

7. Reduced Inflammation: Quality sleep helps to lower inflammatory markers in the body, including those that contribute to skin inflammation. By reducing inflammation, sleep can improve conditions like acne, eczema, and psoriasis.

8. Bright Complexion: Lack of sleep can lead to a dull, lacklustre complexion because insufficient rest affects blood flow and can result in a pale or sallow appearance. Quality sleep helps enhance blood circulation, giving the skin a healthy and radiant glow.

9. Skin Allergies: Sleep deprivation can impact the skin's immune response, making it more prone to allergic reactions and irritations. Adequate sleep supports proper immune function, minimising the risk of skin allergies and sensitivities.

To optimise sleep for better skin health, establish a consistent sleep schedule, create a relaxing bedtime routine, and ensure a sleep-friendly environment. Avoiding caffeine and electronic screens before bed and creating a calm atmosphere can enhance the quality and duration of your sleep.

Remember, managing stress and prioritising adequate sleep are essential for overall well-being, including skin health. Implementing healthy lifestyle habits in these areas can help maintain a vibrant and balanced complexion.

The Importance of Sun Protection and Safe Skin Care Practices

The importance of sun protection and safe skincare practices cannot be overstated when it comes to maintaining healthy and youthful-looking skin. Here's an extensive overview of why these practices are crucial:

1. Sun Protection:

    a. Prevention of Skin Cancer: The primary reason for sun protection is to reduce the risk of skin cancer. Prolonged and unprotected exposure to the sun's harmful UV rays is a leading cause of different types of skin cancer, including melanoma, basal cell carcinoma, and squamous cell carcinoma. Regular use of sunscreen and protective measures significantly reduce the chances of developing these conditions.

b. Minimization of Premature Ageing: The sun's UV rays accelerate the ageing process by breaking down collagen and elastin—the proteins responsible for skin's firmness and elasticity. Over time, this can lead to wrinkles, fine lines, sagging skin, and age spots. Proper sun protection helps minimise sun damage and keeps the skin looking more youthful.

c. Prevention of Sunburns: Sunburns not only cause short-term discomfort but also contribute to long-term damage to the skin. Repeated sunburns can increase the risk of skin cancer and accelerate premature ageing. The use of sunscreen, protective clothing, and seeking shade during peak sun hours helps prevent sunburns and safeguard the skin.

d. Protection from Hyperpigmentation: UV exposure can trigger an overproduction of melanin, leading to dark spots and uneven skin tone. By consistently using sunscreen and avoiding excessive sun exposure, the risk of hyperpigmentation is significantly reduced, promoting a more even complexion.

e. Protection against UV Radiation: The sun emits harmful ultraviolet (UV) radiation that can penetrate the skin and cause damage at a cellular level. UV radiation is categorised into UVA and UVB rays. UVA rays penetrate deeply into the skin, causing long-term damage like photoaging and cell damage, while UVB rays primarily affect the upper layers of the skin, causing sunburn and increasing the risk of skin cancer. Sun protection measures like applying broad-spectrum sunscreen, wearing protective clothing, using sunglasses, and seeking shade during peak hours help minimise the harmful effects of UV radiation.

f. Prevention of Melanoma: Melanoma is a type of skin cancer that often develops due to excessive sun exposure. It is considered the deadliest form of skin cancer, as it can metastasize to other parts of the body. By adopting sun protection practices, such as wearing sunscreen with a high SPF and reapplying it regularly, wearing wide-brimmed hats and sun-protective clothing, and seeking shade, the risk of developing melanoma is significantly reduced.

g. Protection for All Skin Types: Regardless of skin colour or tone, everyone is at risk of sun damage. While individuals with fair skin are more prone to sunburns and skin damage, people with darker skin tones can still experience harmful effects from the sun. They are also at risk of developing skin cancer, albeit at lower rates than individuals with lighter skin. Therefore, sun protection practices should be followed diligently by people of all skin types.

h. Sun Protection All Year Round: Sun protection should not be limited to the summer months or sunny days. UV radiation is present throughout the year, even on cloudy or overcast days. It can also reflect off surfaces like sand, snow, and water, intensifying its harmful effects. Therefore, it is crucial to incorporate sun protection into daily routines, regardless of the weather or season.

2. Safe Skincare Practices:

a. Proper Cleansing: Effective cleansing removes dirt, excess oil, bacteria, and pollutants from the skin, helping to prevent clogged pores, acne breakouts, and skin infections. It is important to choose gentle cleansers suitable for one's skin type and to avoid harsh scrubbing or over-cleansing, as these can strip the skin of its natural moisture balance.

b. Moisturization: A well-hydrated skin barrier is essential for overall skin health. Regular moisturization helps to lock in moisture, maintain skin elasticity, and prevent dryness, which can lead to irritation, flaking, and compromised skin barrier function. Using a moisturiser suitable for one's skin type promotes a healthy, supple complexion.

c. Exfoliation: Gentle exfoliation removes dead skin cells, promoting cell turnover and revealing fresher, smoother skin. Regular exfoliation can improve the texture of the skin, enhance product absorption, and prevent clogged pores. However, it is important to avoid excessive exfoliation, as it can cause irritation and sensitivity.

d. Avoidance of Harmful Ingredients: Safe skincare practices involve being mindful of the ingredients used in skincare products. Avoiding harsh chemicals, fragrances, sulphates, parabens, and other potential irritants helps minimise the risk of skin allergies, inflammation, and adverse reactions.

e. Patch Testing: Before incorporating new skincare products into your routine, it is advisable to perform a patch test. Applying a small amount of the product to a small area of skin and monitoring for any adverse reactions can help identify potential sensitivities or allergies.

f. Prevention of Skin Irritation and Sensitivity: By following safe skincare practices, individuals reduce the risk of skin irritation, redness, and sensitivity. Using products with gentle, non-irritating ingredients, avoiding abrasive scrubs, and using lukewarm water during cleansing can help maintain the skin's natural moisture barrier and prevent damage.

g. Prevention of Acne Breakouts: Proper skin care practices, like regularly cleansing the skin and using non-comedogenic products, can help prevent clogged pores and acne breakouts. This is especially important for individuals with oily or acne-prone skin. Avoiding excessive scrubbing or harsh treatments can prevent irritation and inflammation, which can worsen acne.

h. Maintaining Optimal Skin Hydration: Safe skincare practices, including moisturising, prevent excessive dryness, flakiness, and irritation. A well-hydrated skin barrier acts as a protective shield and promotes healthy-looking skin. Choosing a moisturiser suitable for one's skin type and applying it regularly can enhance skin health and prevent moisture loss.

i. Preservation of Skin's Natural pH Balance: The skin has a slightly acidic pH that acts as a defence mechanism against harmful bacteria and other pathogens. Using gentle cleansers with a pH balance similar to the skin's natural pH helps maintain this protective barrier, preventing disruption and potential issues like dryness, sensitivity, and infection.

j. Prevention of Hyperpigmentation and Uneven Skin Tone: Safe skincare practices, such as sun protection and avoiding excessive sun exposure, are instrumental in preventing the development of hyperpigmentation and promoting a more even skin tone. This is especially important for individuals prone to conditions like melasma or post-inflammatory hyperpigmentation.

k. Promoting Overall Skin Health: Safe skincare practices contribute to the overall health and vitality of the skin. By regularly cleansing, moisturising, and protecting the skin from environmental aggressors, individuals can maintain a healthy skin barrier, which supports the skin's natural functions, including protection against pathogens, regulation of moisture, and proper cell turnover.

l. Boosting Self-Confidence and Well-being: Taking care of the skin through safe skincare practices can boost self-confidence and overall well-being. When the skin looks and feels healthy, individuals tend to feel more comfortable and confident in their own skin, leading to enhanced self-esteem and mental well-being.

m. Regular Skin Checks: Performing regular self-examinations of the skin is crucial for early detection of any unusual moles, growths, or changes in the skin. Prompt detection of potential skin cancers allows for timely intervention and improved outcomes.

n. Professional Dermatological Guidance: Consulting with a dermatologist ensures personalised skincare advice and guidance tailored to an individual's specific needs. They can help design a suitable skincare routine, identify potential skin concerns, and provide necessary treatments, ensuring optimal skin health.

Incorporating sun protection measures and safe skincare practices is essential for promoting overall skin health, preventing skin cancer, minimising premature ageing, and maintaining a vibrant complexion. Incorporating these habits into daily routines and seeking professional guidance when needed will help individuals achieve and maintain healthy, glowing skin throughout their lives.

CONCLUSION

The Glowing Guide: Achieving Beautiful Skin through Holistic Skincare is more than just a skincare manual - it is a comprehensive roadmap to radiant and healthy skin. Through its holistic approach, this book empowers you to understand the interconnectedness of your body, mind, and skin, and provides practical advice on nourishing the skin from within, creating an effective skincare routine, and considering lifestyle factors that impact skin health.

By embracing this holistic approach, you can achieve sustainable and long-lasting results, rather than relying on quick fixes and temporary solutions. You will learn to identify your unique skin type and address specific skin concerns with targeted solutions. You will also discover the role of nutrition and supplements in promoting radiant skin and create a skincare routine tailored to your needs. Through special treatments and a focus on lifestyle factors, you will go beyond skincare products and achieve an overall sense of well-being.

Achieving Sustainable Skin Health and a Glowing Complexion

Achieving sustainable skin health and a glowing complexion requires a holistic approach that combines both internal and external practices. It is not just about the products we use on our skin, but also the choices we make when it comes to our diet, lifestyle, and overall well-being. By adopting a skincare routine that prioritises natural and eco-friendly products, avoiding harmful chemicals, and ensuring proper hydration and nutrition, we can promote the long-term health and vitality of our skin. Furthermore, incorporating stress-reducing activities and taking care of our mental and emotional well-being can have a profound impact on the health of our skin. It is important to remember that achieving sustainable skin health is a journey, and consistency and patience are key. With dedication and a mindful approach, we can achieve a luminous, healthy complexion that not only benefits us but also contributes to a healthier planet.

Final Thoughts and Tips for Your Skincare Journey

Embarking on a skincare journey is a personal and unique experience that requires diligence, patience, and self-care. Throughout this journey, it is important to remember that everyone's skin is different, and what works for one person may not work for another. However, there are some universally beneficial tips to keep in mind.

Firstly, it is crucial to understand the basics of skincare, including moisturising, cleansing, and protecting your skin from the sun. Using products that are suitable for your skin type and avoiding harsh chemicals can help you achieve healthier skin.

Secondly, consistency is key. Developing a daily skincare routine and sticking to it will yield the best results. Skincare is a long-term commitment, and results may not be immediate. However, with time, you will start noticing positive changes in the overall health and appearance of your skin.

Additionally, remember that skin care is not only about what you apply topically but also what you consume and how you live your life. A healthy diet, regular exercise, sufficient sleep, and stress management can greatly contribute to the overall health of your skin.

Lastly, do not hesitate to seek assistance from skincare professionals or dermatologists if you face persistent skin concerns or have specific skincare needs. They can provide personalised advice and recommendations tailored to your unique situation.

In summary, a successful skincare journey requires knowledge, consistency, and a holistic approach. By taking care of your skin both internally and externally, adapting to its needs, and making informed choices, you can achieve healthier, radiant skin that boosts your confidence and overall well-being. Remember, self-care is a lifelong commitment, and investing in your skin health is an investment in yourself.

As you embark on your skincare journey, this guide will equip you with the knowledge, tools, and understanding needed to achieve your skincare goals. With patience and consistency, you will witness the transformation of your complexion and the enhancement of your inner radiance. The Glowing Guide is not just a book to read; it is a skincare companion that will inspire and empower you to embrace a holistic approach and unlock your skin's true potential.

So, as you turn the final page of this book, remember that your skincare journey doesn't end here. Use the knowledge gained from The Glowing Guide to continue making informed choices, actively nourish your skin from within, and prioritise a healthy lifestyle. With dedication and perseverance, you will cultivate sustainable skin health and enjoy a glowing complexion for years to come.

Here's to your radiant skin and the beauty that comes from within. May The Glowing Guide serve as your trusted companion on your lifelong skincare journey.